Life Shifts:
Essays of Hope

Edited by Elizabeth Osta

NFB Publishing
Buffalo, New York

Printed in the United States of America

Life Shifts: Essays of Hope/ Osta, et al- 1st Edition

ISBN: 978-1-088883242

1.Life Shifts. 2. Cancer. 3. Cancer Survival. 4. Essays.
5. Family Resource. 6. Osta.

Cover Image by Ann Kemp Fine Art Photography
For More Information Please visit annkemphotography.com

NFB
<<<>>>
NFB Publishing/Amelia Press
119 Dorchester Road
Buffalo, New York 14213

For more information visit

Nfbpublishing.com

For the Pluta Family
and the doctors, nurses, and staff
of the Pluta Cancer Center,
whose dedication
to patient-centered care
has given hope and healing to so many.

For Gary McIntyre,
whose life on his beloved tractor
and his support of Pluta
through his fundraising and magnificent photography
provided inspiration throughout his days.

The Iris, a symbol of hope and faith,
is drawn by Kitty Forbush, RN, OCN

Table of Contents

Acknowledgements

Special thanks to Helen Pluta and all the Pluta Family who continue to promote the values and vision of Pluta Cancer Center through their tireless work in advocating for funding and services and creating social events that feature patients and their families, celebrating sorrows and successes together.

And to Kitty Forbush, chemo nurse extraordinaire who, along with all the nurses and staff, has shown dedication and devotion unparalleled.

A mighty thanks to those who have contributed their story so that others might find comfort.

Foreword

Leslie F. Algase, MD, FACP

It was in July of 2004, unbeknownst to me, that I became a better doctor. It was our first trip to watch a professional tennis tournament in Toronto and my husband had a bone scan the day before we left to investigate a mass in his shoulder. Just before we left for the tournament, we received the news that the bone scan was positive and that he most likely had a chondrosarcoma (bone cancer). We arrived and despite enjoying the tournament that we had very much looked forward to, we were in a state of shock. The first time we walked out of the stadium it hit us even more. There in front of us was a kiosk selling tickets to next year's tournament. It was a jolt for both of us realizing that we couldn't buy those tickets because next year was no longer something we could plan for right now.

He subsequently had surgery to remove the tumor and bone grafting and very, very slowly over several years we were able to get our future back. Thank heavens he is still well and we have been to many subsequent tennis matches together.

Having gone through my own journey as a spouse and caregiver has helped me to guide my patients through theirs. I understand firsthand the stages they are going through and can partner with them and share more than the medical facts about their cancer. Having survived in my own family helps me to prepare my patients to be survivors and to be grateful for each day we are given.

Elizabeth lives this journey every day as well. With this book, more people will start their journeys with the wisdom and guidance of those who understand.

Introduction

When I learned Peg, a bridge group friend, had breast cancer, my first thought was, "Oh, she's a goner." It was 2006. I was moved by the fact that she would need to be with family in her last days and determined I wouldn't interrupt with any visits or cards. These days were for close relatives. My own fear of cancer kept me from getting close.

Occasionally I asked about her and finally, after a year and a half, with cropped hair and a bright smile, she was back to our group. I listened and watched carefully, feeling guilty that I hadn't made any gestures of support. Should I have? Did they matter? Soon enough, I found out.

In 2008, I was diagnosed with the same dread disease, mostly a woman's scourge. I struggled through the first days, my husband and I welling up with tears together as the diagnosis came that the cancer was more extensive than initially thought. Chemo would come first to shrink the tumor, then surgery, followed by radiation. I thought of Peg. She'd gotten through it, hadn't she? But for how long?

I settled in to my treatments, letting the professionals take over. And I was bolstered daily by cards and calls wishing me well. The same cards and calls I had neglected to give Peg. Glad that her other friends had been there for her, I learned firsthand what support meant. I learned that this diagnosis was not a death sentence but rather an entry to a new world of people called cancer survivors. For as long as we could be.

My treatments and surgery had complications. "This usually doesn't happen," they said. But I struggled through, surrounded by love, laughter, and the Hallmark channel.

It's been ten years since my last treatment. Some details are captured in writings I did at the time. I read of remembered courage summoned, the faith that all would be well. I kept the cards that brought tears and remember the meals that said, "I care, we care," that were delivered when so very needed.

How can I help but be grateful? I'm here, I'm well and I'm finding this way to say thank you, to pay it forward.

This collection of essays come from folks who've had similar experiences. They come with a message of resilience and hope that is heard again and again, its truth like the Holy Grail, quested after by those who follow.

It is sent to those newly diagnosed who tremble in fear, to those continuing in treatment and to those who are settled into being survivors.

It's also sent in remembrance of those loved ones who did not survive, who remain a part of our recovery, their laughter, wisdom and acceptance still leading us forth.

—**Elizabeth Osta**

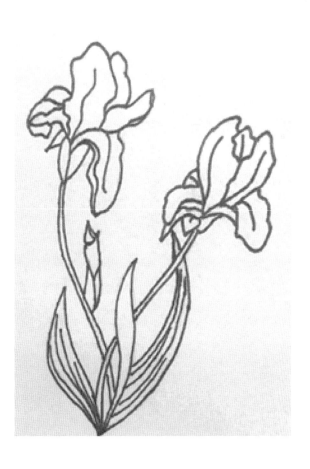

We're all here for a limited amount of time,
and life is difficult - not unfair, but difficult.
The key is to really confront our fears
because when we do,
and when we look at them,
we really begin to realize
that we are capable of handling them.

—Bernie Siegel, M.D.

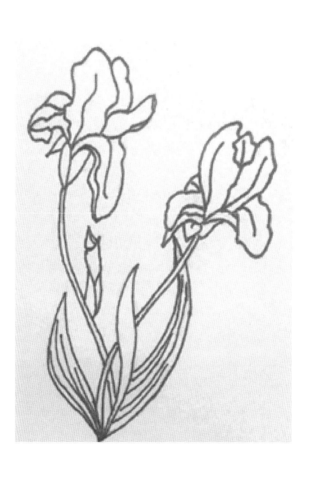

I meandered into middle age with no major medical traumas. So, when endometrial cancer snuck up on me in 2012, I was emotionally ill-prepared, having assumed good health was my rightful reward for a healthy lifestyle. In the long weeks leading up to surgery, a digging anxiety turned me into a soul-less robot at work and a cowardly zombie at home. I knew I wasn't going to die immediately, but the long-range forecast simmered with uncertainty.

Grade 1, Stage 1A, read the pathology report. "Just your garden variety endometrial cancer," said the doctor, excusing me from chemo and radiation. Even the lymphedema that followed remains mild and manageable, though that too sent me into a dark tailspin for months. "Pinky cancer with a hangnail," I finally joked.

Through a support group, I met cancer survivors who had gone through hell and back and seemed far more saddled in courage than I had been. Elsewhere, I studied others who also showed steadiness and resilience in the face of adversity: a kind manager who spent lunch hours visiting a dying spouse at the nursing home; a divorcee who uses a wheelchair who volunteers at a fashion show fundraiser; a sister who danced at the nephew's wedding anyway, knowing the abusive ex-husband was there too.

All these people have become my secret Sherpas, the ones

who teach me that when bad things happen to good people, good people keep living. Eventually, something bad happens to all of us, whether we "deserve" it or not. Nobody gets out of this life alive, right? When that next hardship comes, I want to face it with the graciousness and fortitude of these newfound heroes.

—Karen M.

With my first cancer diagnosis twelve years ago, of esophageal cancer, I had no idea how serious it was and that many did not survive it. I had a lot of faith in my doctors and simply left it in their hands. I had to get accustomed to an entirely new way of eating, radically limiting the amount I could eat at one sitting. When I was told there would be a "new normal" I cynically said "this is a sugar-coated way of saying 'there are some things you'll never do again'". As time went on, I came to believe there is a lot of wisdom in this expression. Just as 'One day at a time' holds significant wisdom, so too did 'new normal' remind me that there was now a major change in my life that I must accept.

With my second cancer diagnosis,(prostate, although 'aggressive' and 'advanced'), my Urologist confidently said "we can CURE this", and that gave me great hope. Radiation was his preferred choice of treatment for men of my age, 78. Treatment was painless, but I was not prepared for the side effects it produced, viz., bowel incontinence, which was devastating and humiliating and which largely kept me captive in my home. But the good news was that the tumor was eliminated, and now, after 4 years, the incontinence is virtually behind me (pun intended).

The major shift in my thinking/feeling following this second bout with cancer was how much to appreciate the everyday pleasures that we normally take for granted, e.g. being able to have a 'normal' bowel movement, on the toilet, WHEN I CHOOSE TO HAVE IT HAPPEN, is a joy many of us never get to appreciate. And of course, the other major shift in my thinking/feeling has been that I am no longer IMMORTAL.

—PJ B

I had "Breast Cancer Lite" eleven years ago. Now time is marked as BBC or ABC – Before Breast Cancer or After! It's unquestionably a mean disease but my only sacrifice was my left breast. Both surgeons (general and plastic) were skilled artists; my primary care doctor gave me her time and asked directly about fears. Fear of death didn't predominate; but I did wonder if I could ever be happy again…

A consultation with an Oncologist at Pluta Cancer Center was complete, complex, kind and reassuring. Since my nodes were negative and my tumor minimally invasive, I could safely choose "no further treatment". That left me with less complicated time to recover, journal, and persist at physical therapy.

Friendship was the greatest learning experience. A "firemen's carry" handed me along with loving gifts and practical problem-solving.

1. – My husband held me when I cried, asked good questions of the care team, emptied drains without being repulsed, and encouraged me to voice thoughts – none being too small or too large! (Ranging from: What about a bathing suit? Does this ruin our plan to grow old together?)

2. – Sons and daughters-in-law who showed up literally and figuratively.

3. – A roster of friends who organized and cooked meals, including some for after I returned to work. Of course
4. – the important things they brought with the food were their open hearts and ears.
5. – Other friends and work colleagues offered prayers, books, chocolate, blankets, expletives(!), and sad observations like "breasts are supposed to be fun!"

To quote Woody Allen, the secret to a good life is "to show up"! This was demonstrated to me and is part of my spiritual practice now. I'm grateful for the scar that reminds me of my good fortune and responsibility to be a thoughtful friend.

—**Theo M.**

I recall three months of sickness: pneumonia, bronchitis, kidney failure, and more. Finally, the diagnosis multiple myeloma was given. My husband and I had the odd feeling of being somewhat relieved. At least now we had something to treat. It was April Fool's Day when the news came. I've found that a sense of humor helps in all situations. Immediately my husband and I went to God for strength and wisdom. Erroneously a doctor who treated me said I had three years to live. It's already more than five. The nurse practitioner told me there is always hope and that hope is sometimes more a cure than anything else. The message from on High never left me, promising me that God would always be with me. My sister, a nurse, advised us well. (Respect the process).

I began treatments, feeling stunned at all the family and people in my life who loved me and cared for and about me. I felt rooted and grounded because God had this in control. I worked with wonderful medical professionals who gave me good care. I went through a lot of testing, treating and tender love. My caretaker husband is amazing. I never knew he could give the support and love he gave and continues to give. Now I receive a check up every eight weeks and take chemotherapy pills for 21 days on and 7 days off. Fatigue is a challenge. I exercise and eat healthy and am strengthened continually by my faith. This experience had shown me a different and, I think, a better perspective of life. I am taking better care of myself (emotionally and physically) and feel cared for. I have returned to work and am living every day in light and love and gratitude.

—**Jane D.**

Those who know me will tell you that I am cautious, often fearful, anxious, and too frequently worried about "what if's". When I was diagnosed with breast cancer last year, something shifted inside of me, and although scared, I suddenly felt a sense of certainty. I was not worried that I would not tolerate chemotherapy, I was not anxious about surgery, and "what if I don't survive this" was not a concern for me. I filled myself with confidence that I was going to be ok. I began each day with prayers for healing, patience, courage, and strength. My relationships with my husband, daughters, family, friends, and most importantly, God, became stronger and deeper than ever. Living my life with a positive outlook despite the detour, was not something temporary for me until I completed treatment-this has been a forever change. Faith and inner peace have replaced fear and worry.

—Cyndi T. (Diagnosed June 2018)

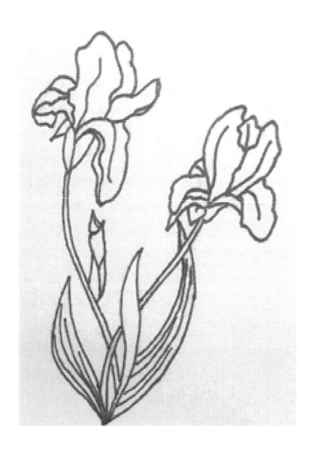

In September of 2012 while on vacation in Sedona, Arizona, I experienced an awful pain in my mid-section. I called my GP back home and he arranged a CT Scan on the day I got home. The pain never reoccurred.

The scan showed a mass on the end of my pancreas and more tests were scheduled – nuclear tests and an MRI. It was decided to remove said mass without a biopsy. My spleen and gall bladder where removed at the same time. The pathology report, which took two weeks to receive, showed no cancer, so no chemo or radiation. This news was wonderful and, because I had lost two friends to pancreatic cancer, I was overjoyed. I knew that pancreatic cancer was pretty much a death sentence.

I was placed on a schedule of MRI's every six months for five years, and thinking I was home free at that mark, I was thrown of a loop when two tumors were on my liver. The doctors theorized that some cancer cells had metastasized to the liver. But they'd told me the mass on my pancreas was NOT cancerous, so how could this be?

I was assigned an oncologist who again set up an MRI every six months and we decided to 'wait and watch" on the liver tumors. So, for the past two years I've been "on hold" = no hormone shots – just 'wait and watch". How do I feel about cheating cancer once and not getting on the medical merry-go-round again?

At first (with the pancreas tumor) I was shocked and sobbed to my brother that I was facing a death sentence. Few escape death when they have pancreatic cancer. After the initial shock, I started picking out my six pall bearers. A typical Irish reaction to bad news – "let's get on with it". I rationalized that I'd had a good and full life and luckily had no children nor a husband to leave behind.

I'd volunteered at a hospice for ten years and realized what "the end" would look and feel like. Not a cheerful thought, but at lease the patients were kept comfortable with drugs. I think of myself as a practical person and so decided I would have to take this news and its repercussions a day at a time. Maybe it was too soon to pick out the dress I would wear at my wake.

It has been two years since the discovery of my liver tumors and I'm still here, aware that my luck may run out some day. But I know that every day going forward is a gift. I have a friend who shares my surgeon and my oncologist at the Wilmot Cancer Center who has a similar track record. He is ten years out. His cancer travelled from the pancreas to the liver (like mine) and then to his lungs. He's gone through chemo and radiation. So as my Sainted Mother would remind me – things could always be worse. There are a lot of people in worse shape than I am so, I should quit whining and "get on with it". That's what I try to do every day. One of my favorite mantras is "worry less and pray more".

—**Rose R.**

It's hard to remember back thirty-five years ago when I was first diagnosed with fourth stage Hodgkin's Lymphoma. I had just buried a friend with second stage Hodgkin's. I had three young children, a terrible marriage and was filled with mind- numbing fear. I ran into a fellow shop owner who gave me the number of her aunt in Ohio who was a fourteen-year survivor of Hodgkin's. She became my hope during my two-year struggle to survive.

When I was asked to write something for this book, I began to think about that time and it brought up so much pain that I choose not to think about. The lessons I learned during my illness are forever consciously carried with me.

I'm am turning seventy-three and my health is good, my life is even better. And I am still learning on this challenging and wonderful journey!

—Cheryl H.K.

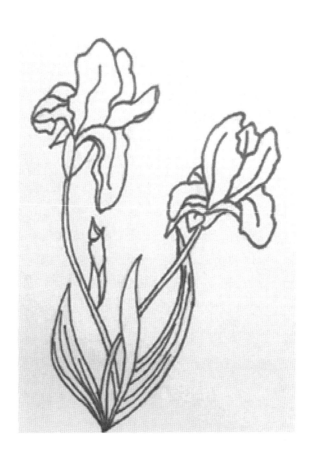

Melanoma was not my first rodeo with cancer. I was diagnosed with Stage 3 prostate cancer in January 1999, at age 51. In January of 2009, at age 61, I was diagnosed with Stage 3b melanoma. Now in January of 2019, I'm 71 years old and fearful of this time period because previous cancers were exactly ten years apart to the month. Although surgery and immunotherapy have given me time, I do not have a completely clean bill of health due to lymph node spread. I am reminded that I need periodic checkups for the rest of my life by my oncologist and dermatologist.

I have greater awareness and appreciation for the life I have been given. I find sweetness in and savor every day and every event. When I get up each morning, I think about this extra time. I notice smaller things in life and appreciate the beauty in them. I'm not as bothered by the mundane issues that throw other people into a tizzy.

My wife and I celebrate sunrises and sunsets almost every day. I have been able to see my children grow into full adulthood and go forward with their lives, which gives me a tremendous amount of joy. I'm living "plus time" with gratitude for all who helped me, especially my loving wife, in every phase.

—**Neil S.**

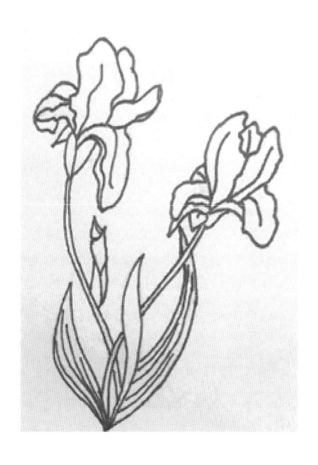

Happy Birthday, you have breast cancer! As I look back on it, this was really the best gift I had ever received. Cancer gave me time to reflect on where I was and where I want to go in this precious life. It helped me realize that even though you take care of yourself by eating well and exercising, it doesn't make you immune to getting a disease like breast cancer. It helped me understand that I had too much stress in my life and that I must reduce this stress for a healthier future. Cancer gave me an opportunity to have closer and more meaningful relationships with family and friends. These wonderful, caring people showed me how to love unconditionally and what it means to truly care for someone. Indeed, the trajectory of my life has shifted because of this unexpected birthday gift for which I will always be grateful.

—Kim R

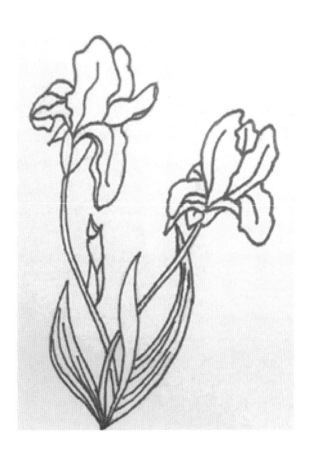

The question asked was "What shifted for you when you were diagnosed with cancer?" For some reason, that is a tough question. In the immediate days following the diagnosis, in May 2007, there was no time to think – it was a whirlwind of different doctor's appointments and decisions to make – reconstruction or not, should I ask for a double mastectomy, what surgeon(s) did I want?

Later, when there WAS time to think, I realized that I was just "along for the ride". Good and bad, all of a sudden there was more attention on me than I was comfortable with... slowly, I realized that for many people, my cancer diagnosis had become my identity. Looking back now, I am aware that in order to not lose my real self, I took on the journey as just another bump in the road of life - no big deal! One friend asked me if in the dark of night, did I worry about death? – honestly, I truly never did. As long as I did everything they told me to do, then I could eventually put this all behind me, my hair would grow back and I could go on with my life, like it never happened.

I am happy to say that is exactly what happened for me. It's not very exciting, or even note-worthy, but in truth not much shifted. I don't keep track of how many years it has been. And weeks or even months go by now, without even a thought of that part of my journey. Am I lucky because of that? Or maybe just blissfully unaware that it could always rear its ugly head again? Maybe, but if it does, I hope I can react the same way!

—**Peg E**

What shifted for me when I was diagnosed with cancer, was my determination to not let cancer define my life. I was looking at my diagnosis as a bump in the road of life and I would look back at it as just that, a really BIG bump in the road. I was not going to let it keep me down. I took six weeks off for recovery from surgery and only a few days off after each chemo treatment, even though my husband wanted me home. Being a patient and employee at Pluta is a blessing in disguise. It shows patients that we can get through this bump in the road with all the love and support of the staff at Pluta.

—**Kelly Z.**

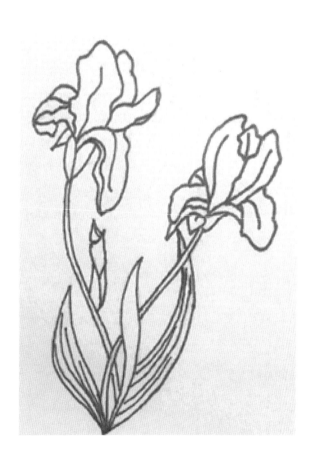

You hear about it. Friends and family members get "the diagnosis." I never thought about it happening to me. But it did and suddenly I found myself swept up into a terrifying whirlwind of medical tests, new doctors, plans for surgery and follow-up treatments. I was about to go on a journey, one that was scary, and with one goal in mind... to heal and survive. Both of which... I did.

What shifted? Everything. The way I thought about life, including how vulnerable we all are. That there is a plan, and we have no idea what it is. I had no idea of the outcome, but I was determined that I was going to do whatever it took to beat the disease. In a short period of time, I shifted from a cancer victim to a cancer fighter to cancer survivor.

—**Susan M.**

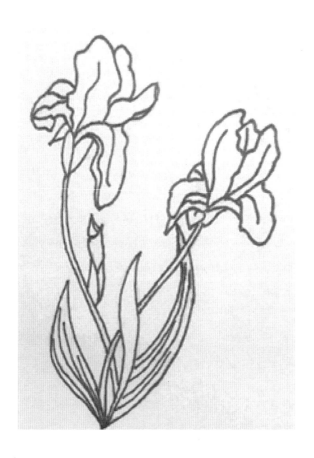

My recollection of dates is a bit foggy but in about 2003 I was diagnosed with prostate cancer. I went through the biopsy testing and confirmed the condition. I was only sixty-five at the time. There were several treatment options available, so we investigated which one seemed most appropriate by talking to five different doctors. We settled on surgery to remove the whole thing.

A follow up visit with the urologist doing a cystoscopy discovered several cancerous polyps in my bladder. These turned out to be unrelated to the prostate cancer. They were also removed.

A few months later, I had a peculiar feeling in my abdomen and through a colonoscopy, discovered colon cancer. The ascending section of my colon was in trouble. It was removed and a course of chemotherapy was started. As it turned out, this cancer was also not related to the other two types of cancer that I had previously. I was to have twelve treatments, but after only 10, neuropathy was showing up, so they stopped the treatments.

Now that I'm 81, the specialists that were treating me feel that I'm free of whatever little things were giving me a hard time. They are gone. Good riddance. It's now time to get on with things I want to do.

—**Pat M.**

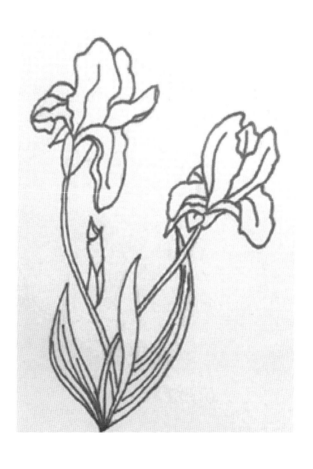

When I was diagnosed with breast cancer, my faith in God helped me to stay calm. I talked to God daily. He answered my questions. I asked God whether I should have both breasts removed. One morning about 3 a.m. I heard this quiet voice say, "Have both removed!" I never questioned it. I trusted. Even though the cancer had been initially found only in the left breast, I had both removed.

After the surgery, the test came back several weeks later. The right breast was precancerous. I was told I made a great call. I can't take the credit. God made the call. I asked God to be with me through surgery and the chemo, and I had no adverse effects from either.

My faith has strengthened. I ask God about all plans. God is good. I am grateful.

—**Lucille B.**

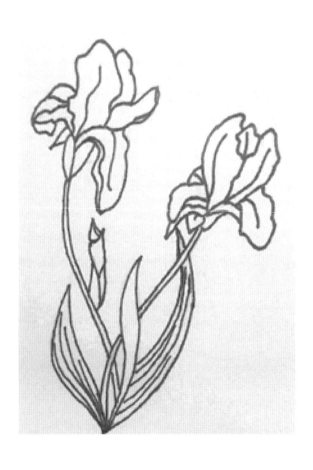

Nobody is ever ready to be told 'you have breast cancer'. After my mother's death at 52 of the dreaded disease, the thought of breast cancer never really left me. When the result of my biopsy came back positive, I was not surprised or shocked.

The day I entered the Pluta Building it really hit me. Throughout my interview I could not stop crying.

The care and emotional support I received made it possible for me to cope with my new reality. I remember finally accepting the fact that it was okay to go shopping for new clothes. A future was possible. Traveling is my way of coping.

I was lucky to have met the wonderful staff at Pluta and brave fellow cancer survivors.

—Helga H

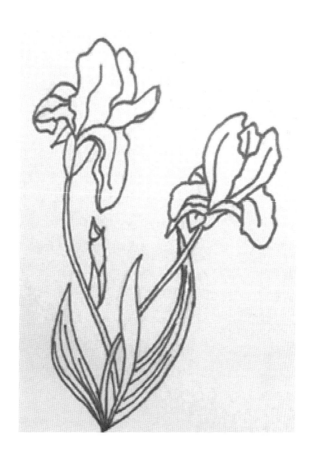

My gynecologist found the lump in my breast during a routine visit; I said, "That wasn't so great." And she said, "That's my job," very matter-of-factly.

She recommended a surgeon who turned out to be wonderful, both personally and as a surgeon: supportive, warm, and an excellent doctor. She (or someone, can't remember who) recommended a book on my kind of cancer. Since I am a bookish person, of course I read it. It is by Robert Bazell and discusses the making of Herceptin, a new treatment for the kind of breast cancer that I had. I am sure (I know) I was anxious about everything, but with the support of friends and family, I went through chemotherapy and Herceptin treatment with only a few glitches, and now, nine years later, I am still enjoying life, reading, and savoring the coming of spring.

I will be eighty-nine in June of this year. So, my life hasn't shifted all that much, unless you count the vicissitudes of old age.

—**Nancy B.**

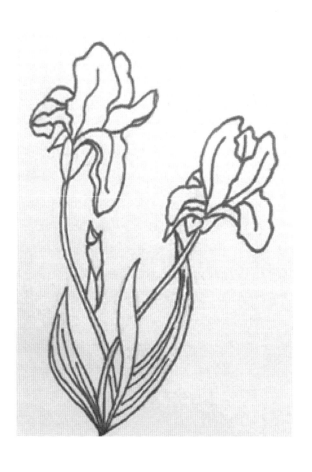

My life changed forever the day before Thanksgiving 2007. I had taken the week off in anticipation of hosting Thanksgiving dinner for family. My screening colonoscopy also happened to be scheduled for that week. I never expected a diagnosis of rectal cancer that day, nor did my doctor! My outlook and perspective on life changed that week and have continued since. Family and friends became the focal point of my life and the motivation to keep fighting. I was blessed to have been referred to Pluta (my angels) and to have a great team taking care of me and guiding me through the "bumps in the road." I have also been blessed with the love and support of family and friends, especially my husband who has been and still is my rock. I now look to my life as a journey with many "new normals" and am thankful every day for all I have been blessed with.

—**Wanda M.**

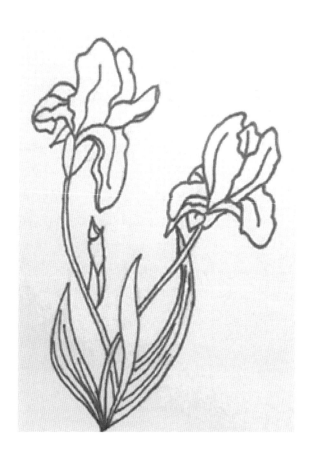

I broke out in hives as my breast was examined for the second time in one appointment. *This can't be good,* I thought! Yet somehow it was good. After the excruciating needles and persistent probing was completed, something shifted. At first, it was imperceptible. Sure, I was grateful to be alive, glad that the partial mastectomy of my right breast was healing, the numbness something I've learned to live with. The lymphedema wasn't anything I bargained for and like the ever-present internet told me, sometimes breast cancer survivors say it's the worst part. But what shifted for me didn't come until a year later. At Christmas time. I cried at the drop of a hat, I was moved by everyone's pain. Like the title of the book that I had recommended to so many, I'd been 'broken open'. I'd begun to feel others' heartaches with an open heart, not a fearful one. I knew for the first time what it meant to have someone reach out to me in compassion. And what I could do in return. It still makes me cry to realize how infrequently we allow ourselves the depth of such connections. And it still makes me grateful to know I've experienced this truth before it was too late!

—**Elizabeth O.**

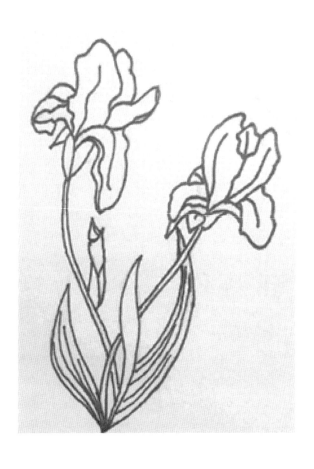

I have made wonderful friends...on this journey and for that I'm grateful. I miss Gary more than I can say and all the other friends I've met along the way. Having survivors guilt I guess.

—**Karen L.**

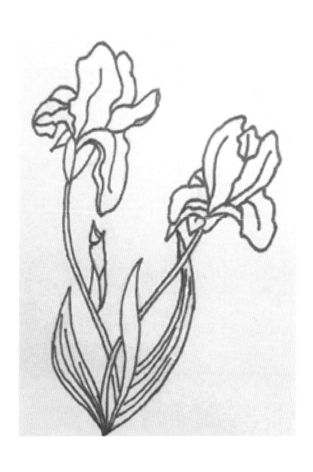

Going through the diagnosis of cancer, or having a loved one who has cancer, can be an overwhelming experience with many different feelings and emotions. There can be sunny thoughts one day and feelings of gloom the next day – or both in the same day – ups and downs like a roller coaster. With the support of caring friends and family, especially those who have been "down the same road," their encouragement can help get us through this part of life's journey. We can come out of this with more compassion and understanding for others who have cancer. Just as someone helped you through your cancer journey, you can one day return that kindness to others.

It seems like my resentment…my anger…my sadness…of having a loved one diagnosed with cancer, and having had cancer myself, gradually shifted to compassion for others who were faced with cancer.

I want you to know I care…about you…and your walk with cancer.

—**Patty L.**

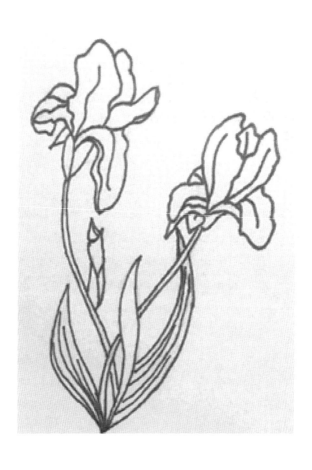

Last year (February 2018), my yearly blood work revealed an elevated PSA. My doctor sent me to a urologist who performed two biopsies before telling me that I had Stage One prostate cancer. He recommended surgery to remove the prostate and said that it was discovered early and the success rate is very high. I was sixty-five years old and hadn't been in the hospital since a tonsillectomy when I was 8 years old. I am a Christian, but also a chronic worrier. I prayed to God that He would help me through this because I cannot do it on my own. No one wants to hear that cancer is in their body. When I first heard the news, I did not have a breakdown, nor did I even cry. I felt the peace of God immediately.

I began reading devotionals about fear and worry, reading through the psalms and praying constantly. I listened to more praise and worship music than I normally did. I learned through the help of the Comforter, the Holy Spirit, to lean on the Almighty Father and trust in Him.

The day that I went in for surgery (August 20th), I had no fear at all. The surgery was successful. And I continue to praise God continually. I understand that many people do not get as hopeful a prognosis as I received, but I will testify that 'God is able to do immeasurably more than all we ask or imagine, according to his power that is at work within us.' Eph. 3:20

—William S.

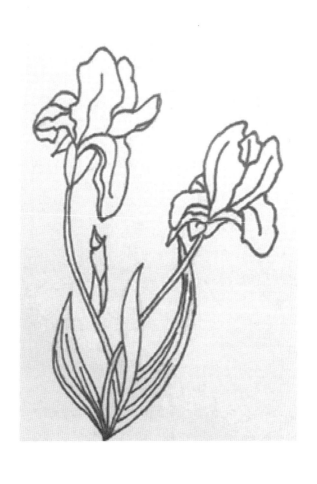

The day cancer changed my life I was waiting for a tour of Gilda's house, the support center built by Gene Wilder in honor of his wife, comedian Gilda Radner, who died from cancer. I was shown to the library where I sat alone for what seemed hours. I was deep into my own pity party as I took stock of my life. My marriage was failing, and my business was losing money. I had a mortgage on the house I was living in and two additional mortgages on rental properties that both needed repairs.

I'd found the lump and went in for the mammogram the Friday before Labor Day weekend. By the end of the day my doctor had called with the news. I had a biopsy Tuesday and a mastectomy the next day.

When I was halfway through chemotherapy and wandering through each day like a zombie, I thought a book might get my mind off my problems for a minute. I scanned the shelves. I pulled out a copy of Excuse Me Your Life is Waiting by Lynn Grabhorn and read the whole thing while I was in the waiting room. The message was simple and beautiful. Get clear about what you want, get out of your own way, and focus on the outcome.

For months I'd made only half-hearted efforts to improve my financial situation. I wasn't taking advantage of the fact that for the first time in my life I had time of my own. I'd been spending my time focused on my problems and hadn't been open to opportunities.

I began to practice the message I'd taken to heart. Less than a month later, I found a buyer for both of my rental properties. Closing out those two mortgages helped me pay down my debt. Shortly after that, my former boss called with a lead on a consulting engagement, and I secured a position on a consulting team that I was uniquely qualified to fill.

But that respite was short lived. I finished the consulting engagement and began to spiral down into depression.

After each outpatient visit to my oncologist, I would stop at the bookstore for coffee and to browse the books before I went home. As I looked through the self-help section, coincidentally, the same book caught my eye. I sat down and started to read it again. I remembered to remember the lesson I'd learned the last time. I bought the book and over my cup of coffee wrote, "By the end of this month I will be hired for another consulting engagement."

As I was leaving the bookstore I received a call from the Chief Operating Officer of a consulting firm who remembered a vignette I shared with him regarding one of the assignments I had early in my Army career. He was checking my availability to staff a consulting engagement that needed someone with that experience. A few days later I was on my way to New York for that engagement. My life hasn't had to wait for me since.

—**Leah L.**

At age 85 years, I was diagnosed with non-Hodgkin's Lymphoma, cancer of the lymph nodes. The body has a network of about 500 lymph nodes mainly located in the soft tissue, but some are attached to the organs, such as the liver. A malignant tumor under my chin was surgically removed and I was regularly monitored at The Pluta Cancer Center.

Many cancers, excluding those of genetic origin, are the result of exposure or activities that one experienced many years earlier.

From June 1948-July 1951 I was employed at the Manhattan Project of the Atomic Energy Commission working with radioactive chemicals. There were no precautions or protections taken to shield the radiation while I was there.

My life shift is to urge everyone to protect themselves from practices that might cause cancer or other medical conditions in later life. This includes over exposure to the sun (since the ozone layer is compromised), exposure to pesticides, herbicides, pollutants in drinking water, foods, air (any source of smoke), removal of asbestos, industrial residues of unknown nature and numerous other contaminates. I urge that this protection begins as early as possible.

—June Stornelli

Hope is the thing
with feathers
that perches in the soul –
and sings the tunes
without the words –
and never stops at all.

—Emily Dickinson

Essays
from Caregivers

Love recognizes no barriers.
It jumps hurdles,
leaps fences,
penetrates walls
 to arrive at its destination
full of hope.

—Maya Angelou

Elizabeth always hated mammograms. She spoke of dense breast tissue and having her boob slammed in a refrigerator door. I was thankful that guys didn't have to go through that.

That day she came home in a grim mood: retakes, waiting for a diagnosis. This was followed by a call; invasive ductal carcinoma – CANCER. My first thought was "Am I going to lose another wife?" My first wife had died from diabetes complications some thirty-two years before, leaving me with two small children. Elizabeth had come along to bring love back into my life.

Right away I thought of three acquaintances, Ginger, Lillian, and Sheila, who had died from breast cancer, and then there was Elizabeth's aunt, Sister Betty, who died at age 83, having put off seeing a doctor until it was too late for treatment.

Elizabeth jumped in to organize her treatment. We immediately began learning lots of medical stuff; Stage 2, sentinel node, mastectomy versus lumpectomy, breast reconstruction, chemotherapy, radiation. The oncologist at Pluta Cancer Center assured us that breast cancer was, at this point, a chronic, treatable disease with a reasonable chance of survival. The treatments weren't pretty but usually successful. Hair loss was "when", not "if".

During the next two years of talking with surgeons and

oncologists, support groups, sitting with Elizabeth in the chemo room, waiting during surgery, a port "gone South", and wigs, I remained confident that WE were going to get through it.

As the years have passed, I have realized how much this journey has brought us together, with lymphedema a daily reminder. The TV ads for Metastatic Breast Cancer drugs remind me how important it is to make each day count.

—**Dave V.**

As a caregiver, no matter how I felt on the inside or the outside, I always had to be positive, encouraging, helpful, and available for the smallest need. I knew the seriousness of cancer and the need for support. A cancer diagnosis changes everything.

I learned so much being part of a cancer support group at Pluta. At first, I thought it would be a 'downer,' but just the opposite happened. I gained so much from others; it gave me strength to be a caregiver.

As soon as my wife felt better, we started traveling, and our trips together have helped us cope.

—John H

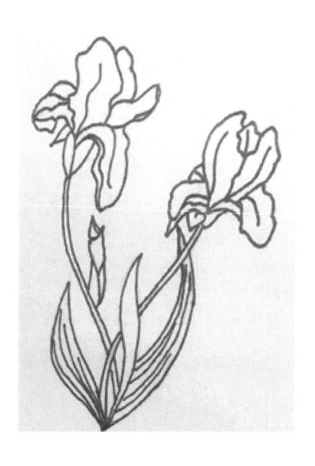

When one of my owners suffered from cancer I knew something was wrong. I did my best to provide love. I found laying my head on her lap provided comfort and distraction from worry. Our routine had to change. I missed our walks together.

—**Bandit H, beloved dog**

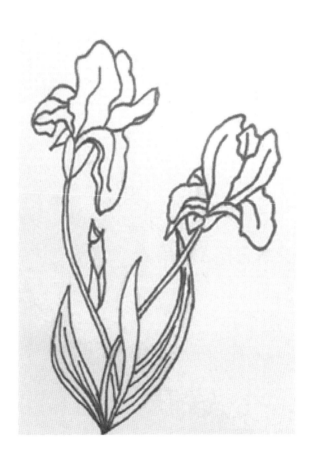

People rarely think of cancer therapy as a pleasant experience, which makes us an exception. My wife Jane M. has been contending with breast cancer periodically for over twenty years, with treatment being primarily lumpectomies. Having recently moved to Rochester, the 2018 treatment changed to a lumpectomy plus extended radiation therapy at the Pluta Cancer Center.

With some trepidation, we went to her first treatment at the center. We did not expect to be in a warm, comfortable setting, but that was exactly what we found. Everyone exuded confidence; all were upbeat – even the receptionist. We agreed that if you are going to have cancer treatment, this is the place to have it. The entire experience was comforting, like being surrounded by family. The long drive to get there turned always to the expectation that the outcome would be favorable. We were not disappointed.

We will not forget the last days of her treatments, when two of the nurses escorted Jane to the 'bell' that marked the end of her radiation therapy. The bell rang loud and clear. She was rid of her cancer. The staff seemed genuinely pleased that Jane had successfully completed her radiation program, her cancer was gone. They gave her a big hug and sent her on her way.

Surrounded by optimism, it was a triumph for all of us, physically and emotionally. From start to finish, we could not have had a more pleasant medical experience.

— **Verner M.**

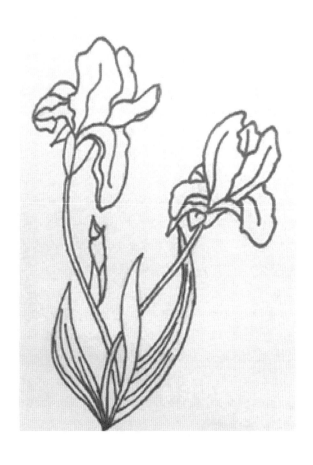

Our relationship is about mutual caring so it was easy except for the scary part! The "C word" as we used to say. His former doctor didn't believe in "those" tests so Pat never had any. There was a very slight symptom and off we went to a new doctor who did believe... The outcome was positive and we checked with four more doctors.

As treatments began there were more tests and other cancers. None related to the others. More treatments more tests.

Nothing else in our lives was as important as improved health and survival. However, that isn't the way we spoke to one another.

It was our work, our jobs, keeping track, three colors of ink for the different treatments with different cancers and doctors.

Other activities and issues dropped away. The blessing of free parking right outside the clinic door, volunteers with goodies in their pockets during chemo. Old friends emerged from nowhere to bring a sandwich so I could go out. Shared advice from survivors.

Twelve chemo treatments were prescribed but after ten his body could take no more. The oncologist and neurologist agreed. Fifteen years later the peripheral neuropathy lingers but health prevails!

Visits to the doctors have lessened. Now they say "you don't need to come in every year". Every five years is enough. But not when your mother, brother, and sister have all died from the disease. We are ever vigilant. We are ever loving and grateful as well!

—**Margaret C.**

My sister Diane was diagnosed with Stage 1 breast cancer. I went cold with worry, never thinking that would happen to our family. When it advanced to Stage 4, it rocked my world! My sister, my best friend, will probably die. I was not sure what I would do without her.

She lived for five years. Very soon after her passing my only other sister Linda was diagnosed with Stage 1 ovarian cancer. I wondered, "Why was I saved from this insidious disease?" I have always taken very good care of myself, but now I started eating better and doing more exercise. Thankfully Linda is doing wonderfully well after five years. I spend more time with her, we travel together and soak up life together, as we are very aware of how precious life is.

When Linda had her hysterectomy, the surgeon cut her bowel—she almost died! I became her care giver, something I never thought I knew how to be. It seemed to come naturally. Maybe it does when you love someone so much.

I still feel such a loss without Diane in my life. No more daily calls, no more sister bonding. Yet I feel blessed that I had so many years with her; I am now a mother figure to her two wonderful daughters and their families, as well as keeping in touch with her grieving husband, who has connected with a high school sweetheart as his wife suggested during their last days together.

—Jeanne M

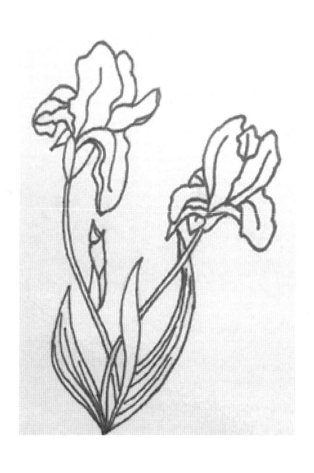

Y OUR HUSBAND HAS CANCER!!!! These were words I
never thought I would hear, but twelve years ago I heard them
as PJ was diagnosed with esophageal cancer. His surgeon is well
known in Rochester, New York and is considered THE BEST!!!
I had complete faith that the surgery would be successful and
that PJ would recover. I was right. We had to completely adjust
our eating habits and choice of food. It was a challenge, but one I
was capable of doing. As long as I have the facts and am told the
truth, I believe I am able to do what I need to do.

Eight years later, I heard the words YOUR HUSBAND HAS
PROSTATE CANCER!!!! Even though the cancer was "aggressive
and advanced", the urologist said "We can cure this." Again, I
believed and trusted the urologist because he was one of the best
in Rochester. PJ and I were in our late 70's so intercourse wasn't a
huge part of our lives. Now, I knew it would be even less.

Now we have been told that PJ is cancer free. We recently
traveled to Tucson, Arizona for seven weeks. Our life goes forward and we are living it "One Day at a Time."

—**Sandy B.**

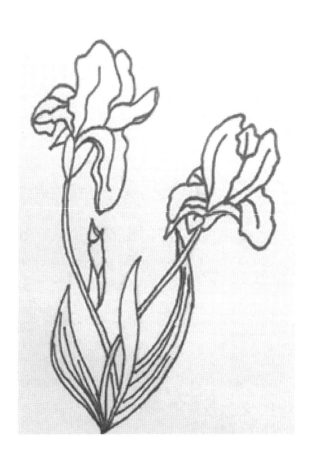

When my husband completed surgeries for Stage 3b melanoma, I was asked to accompany him every day for IV interferon immunotherapy for six weeks. I was overcome with fear. I did not have vacation time, and he was not able to work. Thankfully, both of our employers gave us the time and compensation, so I was able to shift to caretaker without reservation.

After his first treatment, he experienced high fever, chills, and anxiety most of that night. There was no doubt that I needed to shift into high alert and monitor him all night. It was no coincidence that my focus changed from "worry" to "one minute at a time." In that six weeks, I learned how to take care of him and myself. While he received treatments, he dozed, so I walked to a park nearby. I began to see goodness everywhere, in the blades of grass, flowers, people and pathways. I let my body guide me during these walks, to see different paths and people. I became more open to really seeing people, looking in their eyes and greeting them.

When Neil was able to receive immunotherapy injections at home, I returned to work. Wearing work "like a loose garment," I shifted from a type-A personality to taking each day as it was. When I returned home, if Neil felt up to it, we would go for a short drive in the car. Again, I saw the good in people, places, and things everywhere. It was like my higher power nudging me to get out of my self-absorption and really notice what is. To this day, we still look forward to drives, especially in the afternoons, just before sunset (or moonrise). When I slip back into self-absorption, I remember this time and get called back to the goodness around all of us.

—**Karen S.**

In April 1996 my spouse of twenty-two years, Brita, was diagnosed with ovarian cancer. Two years later, in April 1998, she died. There were many things that shifted for both of us when we learned the news and as the disease and the treatments took their course. It seemed that Brita's life took on a grace during those two years that I had not seen in her before. She became amazingly compassionate toward herself, me, and others. And both of us found increased joy in "simple" things—nature, friends and family, beauty, mindfulness.

For me, one of the most profound shifts was related to my fear of death. During a time when we both believed death was imminent for Brita—though that didn't turn out to be the case until later—we both felt a surprising sense of acceptance and peace. We had both been fighting this disease with all we had, and yet during those moments we were ready for death to come. Then those moments passed and the life force returned and we again gave all we had to the fight. But I came away with the belief that when the time of death does come for me, as it did for Brita, there will be a peace that comes with it, and that thought has brought me much comfort.

Another shift for me was that Brita's illness started me on a search for spiritual grounding that led me first to Buddhist meditation practice and later, as the years passed, into seminary and ministry, which has included hospital chaplaincy and work with grief groups. It's been over twenty years now since she died. At the time I felt like my own life was over too, but today my life is fuller than I could ever have imagined.

—**Peggy M.**

Optimism is the faith
that leads to achievement.
Nothing can be done
without hope and confidence.
—Helen Keller

Life Shifts
An Afterword

For thirty-five years I have been honored to bear witness to the incredible courage, faith and determination shown by my patients, including those who lost the battle.

As an oncology infusion nurse at Pluta Cancer Center, I have been made a better human being for I've been graced with the trust from patients to guide them, to cry with them, to listen to them, to sing with them, to laugh with them, to teach them, to let them be however they need to be. It's thrilling to see someone's fear melt away and be replaced with the belief that they can do this.

I often say in my work, I get to live the Golden Rule:
DO UNTO OTHERS AS YOU WOULD HAVE THEM DO UNTO YOU.

The words in this powerful little book are the heartfelt stories of many who have endured their cancer diagnosis and treatment and are now embracing survivorship. Their caregivers give powerful testimony as well. So scary at first yet somehow it becomes a road of acceptance, an acknowledgement of personal power and ultimately a celebration of life's joys and a greater appreciation of the sweetness of life on life's terms.

I salute you all. You are all my heroes.

With love,

Kitty Forbush, RN,OCN